Detox Formula

Concise Solution on How to Naturally Detoxify

Your Liver, Kidney, and Blood for Reversing

Diabetes and High Blood Pressure

Bill Sam

Copyright © 2019 Bill Sam

All rights reserved. No part of this publication may be reproduced, distributed, or transmitted in any form or by any means, including photocopying, recording, or other electronic or mechanical methods, without the prior written permission of the publisher, except in the case of brief quotations embodied in critical reviews and specific other non-commercial uses permitted by copyright law.

ISBN: 978-1-63750-192-4

Table of Contents

DETOX FORMULA 1

INTRODUCTION 5

CHAPTER 1 8

    LIVER CLEANSING FOODS AND NATURAL HERBS FOR WELLNESS AND FITNESS 8

    DANDELION (TARAXACUM OFFICINALE) 8
        Uses and its Function 9
        How to use Dandelion effectively 10
        Dandelion Remedies 10
    MILK THISTLE (SILYBUM MARIANUM) 12
        Uses and its Function 13
        How to use Milk Thistle effectively 14
        Milk Thistle Remedies 14
    FUMITORY (FUMARIA OFFICINALIS) 16
        Uses and its Function 16
        How to use Fumitory effectively 17
        Fumitory Remedies 18
    CHICORY (CICHORIUM INTYBUS) 19
        Uses and its Functions 19
        How to use Chicory effectively 20
        Chicory Remedies 21
    BOLDO (PEUMUS BOLDUS) 22
        Uses and its Function? 22
        How to use Boldo effectively 23
        Boldo Remedies 23
    ARTICHOKE (CYNARA SCOLYMUS) 25
        Uses and Function of Artichoke 25
        How to use Artichokes effectively 26
        Artichokes Remedies 27

CHAPTER 2 29

    6 HERBS TO IMPROVE KIDNEY AND LIVER FUNCTION NATURALLY 29

CHAPTER 6 45

HOW TO DETOX YOUR BLOOD 45
WHAT TO KNOW BEFORE TAKING ANY HERB 47
SAFEGUARDING YOUR LIVER 51
5 FAIL-PROOF HERBS FOR DETOXIFYING BLOOD NATURALLY & THEIR
PREPARATIONS 54

Introduction

Have you thought of focusing on one facet of your well-being to transform all the other aspects of your wellness-- and simultaneously prevent health problems you didn't even know were lurking beneath the surface?

Detox formula is a clear-cut, effective, wholesome detox plan that will cleanse your liver kidney and blood, which would automatically reset your body and your habits! Tens of thousands of people have already used this groundbreaking guide to rescue ther liver, kidney and blood from life-wasting toxins. Now it's your turn!

In today's world, we have no slight idea of how many symptoms, conditions, and diseases are rooted in an overloaded liver, kidney, blood, and lungs. It's not only about liver cancer, hepatitis, and cirrhosis. Nearly every challenge--from pesky general health issues, to emotional imbalance, to weight gain, to high blood pressure, to heart problems, to brain fog, to skin conditions, to digestive issues and complaints, to autoimmune and other chronic illnesses--has their source and origin in an overloaded liver, kidney, lungs and blood, which can improve and heal when you take good advantage of the knowledge in this book to rejuvenate your organ.

The cause of illness is poison (acidosis), i.e., toxins from our food, water and air. No genuine healing can proceed in such a toxified environment. These book is to treat the cause of illness, not the symptoms! The Detox Formula Sourcebook shows you how to use raw foods and herbs as of the primary means of detoxification, healing, and ultimate regeneration of weak or diseased cells.

This book is hugely helpful for: being clearer-headed, more peaceful, happier, and better able to adapt to our fast-changing times. After reading this book, and making use of the explained information, You will learn how to sleep well, balance blood sugar, lower blood pressure, lose weight, and look and feel younger. A healthy liver, kidney, lungs, and blood are the ultimate de-stressor, anti-aging ally, and safeguard against a threatening world--if we give it the right support in the natural way.

Chapter 1

Liver Cleansing Foods and Natural Herbs for Wellness and Fitness

Dandelion (Taraxacum officinale)

Dandelion-liver-cleansing-food is weed-like plants that grows wildly through the world and two times as a robust liver cleansing food and herb, making great improvements to salads and juices and are plentiful at most marketplaces.

It is an extremely common flower that has many beneficial health properties, but it is mostly called a regular *"weed."* Its fresh leaves can be consumed in salads, and their great purifying power makes dandelion an important component in detoxifying cleanses. *It really is a great ally for liver organ and kidney health, but additionally it is essential in weight loss due to its low caloric content and satiating impact.*

Uses and its Function

It's very good for the liver organ because it raises bile creation (choleretic) and facilitates emptying of the gallbladder (cholagogue). *This makes it one of the most beneficial plant life for liver organ disorders and gallbladder breakdown. It also has the capacity to activate the appetite, help digestive function, and exert a slight laxative impact for avoiding constipation.* It can be used orally as natural tea, fresh salad, or several tablespoons of fresh juice before foods, they have a diuretic and cleaning impact, which is strongly suggested for preventing fluid retention and for eliminating calcium mineral oxalate crystals to avoid kidney stone. This, as well as its important work in assisting the liver organ, makes it a highly effective treatment against *eczema, rashes*, which are generally triggered by autointoxication. *Dandelion is often suggested when months are changing. It is a highly effective treatment for overeating, rendering it helpful for weight control.* Furthermore, *it externally acting as a poultice , helps heal wounds and bruises.*

How to use Dandelion effectively

Its freshly picked leaves may be used to make a fresh juice, utilizing a blender, and then put into a salad. If you fail to obtain it fresh, it is available as troches (dried out) or in teabags, ready for planning infusions and decoctions; it can be purchased in (1/2 to at least one 1 teaspoon [2 to 5 milliliters] every 8 hours), water removed (3/4 to 2 teaspoons [4 to 10 milliliters] every 8 hours), and pills (powdered or dried out).

Dandelion Remedies

By Itself

Digestive and liver organ cleansing infusion: put in a teaspoon of dandelion to a glass of boiling water. Allow it steep for ten minutes and cool. Drink 3 mugs per day, around 30 minutes before foods. *This treatment not only supports digestive function, but it cleanses the whole body.*

Combined

Hepatoprotective and diuretic infusion: mix identical parts liver purifying foods boldo, artichoke, dandelion, and peppermint. Put in a teaspoon of the mix to a glass of boiling water and allow it steep for ten minutes. Serve it and drink it before foods. *It can aid good digestion and facilitate excretion of waste materials substances.*

Mindful Lifestyle Recommendations

organic-dandelion-root-capsules Oregon's Crazy Harvest Organic Dandelion Root

Oregon's Crazy Harvest offers a 100% real dandelion root natural powder for easy absorption and usage of the powerful liver cleaning food. 100% vegan tablets deliver the dandelion natural powder easily to avoid its bitter flavor for individuals who don't like herbal supplements.

Milk thistle (Silybum marianum)

Milk thistle liver-cleansing herb milk is a healthy liver cleansing food and natural herb that grows wild throughout the united states and Europe.

Thistle is local to Mediterranean temperate areas, where it's been used since ancient times. In lots of locations, it is a normal winter vegetable offered at Christmas celebrations. They have a delicate, nice, and somewhat bitter flavor. Though it is not so rich in nutrition, it offers other energetic components, such as *silymarin and inulin*, to which it owes its therapeutic properties.

Uses and its Function

It is one of the very most effective remedies for protecting and recovery the liver organ since it contains silymarin, a material with the capacity of regenerating liver organ cell damaged by harmful toxins and relieving liver organ tissue inflammation. **Milk Thistle** is, therefore, a great treatment for *hepatitis and liver organ failure*. Additionally it is used to take care of liver organ disorders triggered by inadequate bile secretion, such as gallstones and biliary dyspepsia. They have good hepatoprotective results to alleviate symptoms related to overeating and alcoholic beverages and substance abuse. As though this wasn't enough, thistle also stimulates hunger; it is diuretic, has a moderate laxative impact, and helps reduce raised cholesterol levels since it has lipid-lowering activity. Furthermore, *it could be used externally as an anti-inflammatory to alleviate sunburn and dermatitis.*

How to use Milk Thistle effectively

It is available in tinctures (1/4 to 1/2 teaspoon [1 to 2 milliliters] every 8 hours), water removes (20 to 30 drops, 2 or 3 (three times each day)), and dried and surface for preparing infusions. It is pulverized into capsules whose dosage is indicated by the product manufacturer. Moreover, *silymarin is extracted from the fruits of milk thistle, which is an ingredient in multiple liver medications.*

Milk Thistle Remedies

By Itself

Decoction to keep up a healthy liver organ: put in a

teaspoon. 5 of thistle to a glass of water and boil it for 2 minutes. Allow it steep for 5 minutes and cool. Drink 2 or 3 mugs a day before foods for good liver organ function.

Combined

Hepatoprotective tea: Mix similar parts liver cleaning foods milk thistle, rosemary, and boldo. Put in a teaspoon of the blend to a glass of boiling water, and allow it steep for ten minutes. Serve it and drink it before foods. *This tea helps to relieve the liver organ after overeating.*

Mindful Lifestyle Recommends

organic-milk-thistle-extract-capsules Omnibiotics Organic Milk Thistle Extract

Omnibiotics offers higher strength, concentrated 4:1 milk thistle draw out in a vegetarian capsule, free from synthetic elements and poor binders. Concentrated in glutathione revitalizing silymarin for maximum liver organ cleaning and hepatoprotective properties.

Fumitory (Fumaria officinalis)

Fumitory-liver-cleanse sacred, somewhat mystical liver organ cleansing herb which has a quantity of beneficial results on your body.

The term *"fumitory"* originates from the Latin *fumus* ("smoke"), though it is as yet not known whether it's since when it is crushed it certainly makes you cry just like smoke does, or because its leaves resemble the smoke from a fire. Actually, old sorcerers believed that whenever this plant was set burning, its smoke would drive away evil spirits.

Uses and its Function

They have antispasmodic, diuretic, and cleansing properties, but what sticks out most is its capability to promote clean gallbladder function, from its cholagogue and choleretic impact, significantly enhancing the digestive process. *Fumitory is suggested to reduce heavy and difficult digestions, migraine headaches, and intestinal spasms. Used externally, it is a good emollient for reducing eczema and rashes.*

How to use Fumitory effectively

Collect it in the open, then dried out in the color, and retain in tightly shut glass containers, from light. You'll find it in troches (dried out and surface), ready to make tea. Additionally it is possible to buy it as liquid or dry draw out and in pills, the second option being the most useful because its dose, signs, and expiration day are specified by the product manufacturer.

Fumitory Remedies

By Itself

Digestive infusion: add 1 teaspoon of fumitory to a cup of water. Allow it steep for ten minutes and cool. You can sweeten it with honey or glucose, and then drink 3 mugs each day before meals.

Combined

Natural tea for gallstones: mix equivalent parts liver purifying foods and herbs boldo, dandelion, peppermint, and fumitory. Place a teaspoon of the combination into a glass and add boiling water. Allow it steep for ten minutes and cool. Drink 3 mugs per day to digest fat and remove harmful toxins, for dealing with gallstones.

Chicory (Cichorium intybus)

This liver cleansing plant has popularized vegetables such as escarole or endive. *Its leaves are used for both cooking and therapeutic purposes.* Furthermore, *it's dried out root can be considered a healthy espresso substitute.* As a vegetable, it's very easy to get it ready and set with other foodstuffs that counteract its particular bitter flavor to make delicious and relaxing salads with dietary and therapeutic properties.

Uses and its Functions

Whether fresh or dried out, use it before meals. Its components help stimulate the urge for food of children and adults, and fortify the digestive system. Because of its lactucopicrin, accountable for the bitter flavor of chicory leaves, it also offers a cholagogue impact; that is, it facilitates emptying the gall bladder and for that reason, improves food digestive function. Thus, it clears the liver organ and boosts its functions. Chicory is preferred for those experiencing gallbladder and liver organ disorders and slow digestion.

Its mild laxative action also goodies chronic constipation, and its mild diuretic impact helps prevent fluid retention. Dried out chicory root is used as an espresso substitute, with the benefit that it's a digestive infusion with no stimulants.

How to use Chicory effectively

Use its freshly selected leaves in salads or fresh juice. Its juice is very bitter but quite effective for stimulating hunger. Use it's fresh or dried out root for planning decoctions (2 teaspoons per glass). The main is also available dried out and smashed for preparing espresso substitute (dried out, roasted, and natural). It may also be in liquid draw out form (2 to 6 drops each day put into multiple dosages).

Chicory Remedies

Digestive decoction: mix a cup of water with two teaspoons of chicory main and boil it for five minutes. Allow it to steep for 10 minutes and cool. Drink up to 3 mugs each day, before food, to excite your urge for food and to aid digestion.

Mindful Lifestyle Recommendations

1. Roasted-chicory-root, Starwest Wildcrafted Roasted Chicory Main Granules

Starwest offers superior quality, wildcrafted chicory main granules conveniently roasted for easy of use in making teas and decoctions for liver organ cleansing. **Starwest** *is one of the planets esteemed suppliers of organic and* *wildcrafted natural herbs*. Preferences great and simple to use.

Boldo (Peumus boldus)

The native folks of Chile, in the Andes, used ***boldo leaves*** as a *treatment for belly and digestion disorders*. Today, it is an extremely common treatment in pharmacies and health food stores. It is one of the most widely used therapeutic vegetation for pharmaceuticals that treat gallbladder disorders.

Uses and its Function?

This remedy's most significant virtues are its ability to safeguard the liver and its *effectiveness in increasing the production of bile in the liver (choleretic effect) and also to facilitate emptying of the gallbladder (cholagogue effect)*. Boldo leaves are specially recommended for issues with gallbladder function, such as gradual or difficult digestive function, bloating, and bad flavor in the mouth area (bitterness), triggered by malfunctioning gallbladder. Furthermore, *it is a mild yet effective laxative that helps battle chronic constipation.*

How to use Boldo effectively

Mostly, dried and chopped boldo leaves are used for preparing infusions (one teaspoon per glass). Nonetheless it is frequently coupled with other choleretic and cholagogue plant life or laxatives. Additionally, it is sold in tablets in dosages suggested by the product manufacturer. Furthermore, its substances are extracted from boldo bark and found in certain pharmaceuticals for treating liver organ and gallbladder diseases.

Boldo Remedies

By Itself

Infusion for biliary dyspepsia: place a teaspoon of

leaves in a glass of boiling water. Allow it steep for ten minutes and cool. Take 3 mugs per day, around 30 minutes before meals.

Combined

Liver organ decongestant tea: blend equal parts liver organ cleansing herbal remedies boldo, fumitory, rosemary, dandelion, and anise. Place two teaspoons of the combination in a glass of boiling water. Allow it steep for ten minutes and cool. To improve liver organ function, take up to 3 mugs before meals.

Mindful Lifestyle Recommendations

wildcrafted-boldo-tinctureAmazon Therapeutics Organic Boldo Tincture

This ultra-high quality organic, bold extract is within tincture form for easy consumption. Sourced from the vegetation native areas in the mountains of Chile and Peru, *Therapeutics Boldo tincture* is a robust natural medication for safeguarding and cleaning the liver organ. Full-spectrum draws out for maximum effectiveness.

Artichoke (Cynara scolymus)

Although previously it was not given much importance as a therapeutic herb, from the twentieth century on, they have begun to take pleasure from a reputation as a treatment for liver organ cleansing and biliary disorders. A few of its substances are contained in pharmaceutical products for liver organ health.

Uses and Function of Artichoke

Both its leaves and stem, whether fresh or dried, are a great treatment for liver damage and biliary diseases, besides being hepatoprotective (e.g, it protects the liver from toxins). *It is cholagogue and choleretic, which promotes good digestive functions.*

It is an extremely recommended treatment for slow digestive function and liver failing. Additionally, it is diuretic, purifying, and plays a part in the removal of urea, so that it is effective for those experiencing kidney failing. *Artichoke also helps lower blood cholesterol levels.*

How to use Artichokes effectively

The most frequent way of benefiting from its medicinal properties is by consuming fresh artichoke heads. Besides eating artichokes, you can prepare fresh juice using fresh leaves; drink it immediately, because you can only keep it for a couple of hours. To make infusion (1 teaspoon per glass) you can find its leaves, dried and chopped. Use it in tincture (1 teaspoon [6 milliliters] every 8 hours), ampoules (with the liquid remove), and pills (dried out artichoke or draw out powder).

Artichokes Remedies

By Itself

- <u>*Infusion for proper digestive function*</u>: put in a teaspoon of leaves to a glass of boiling water. Allow it steep for ten minutes and cool. Drink it around 30 minutes before meals. It could be sweetened with sugar or honey.

Combined

Regulatory hepatic infusion: mix equivalent elements of the liver organ cleansing herbal products *boldo, artichoke, and thistle*. Blend a teaspoon of the mixture per glass of boiling water and allow it steep for ten minutes. Then serve it and drink three mugs a day, around 30 minutes before meals.

Mindful Lifestyle Recommendations

wildcrafted-artichoke-capsules, Paradise Herbal products Artichoke Extract

Paradise Herbs provides an ultra high quality; full range artichoke leaf removes growth without the utilization of any chemicals and pesticides. Their special low heat removal process preserves all delicate liver cleansing therapeutic compounds just like nature intended.

Chapter 2

6 Herbs to improve Kidney and Liver Function Naturally

Milk Thistle

This herb has been found in medicine for a large number of years. The information shows first hundred years of Romans utilizing it for liver organ health. The active component that helps our kidneys and liver organ is named *silymarin*.

What Does Milk Thistle Do For The Kidneys?

Silymarin can help our kidney cells recuperate faster when it's been subjected to damaging chemicals.

Milk thistle also offers flavonoids, is filled with antioxidants, and will help you produce more of your antioxidants. **Milk thistle** really helps to increase the manifestation of genes involved with generating three of your powerful antioxidants in the kidneys:

- *Glutathione.*

- *Superoxide Dismutase.*

- *Catalase (5)*

Milk thistle also helps to reduce inflammation in our kidneys and could even help protect you from kidney malignancy. *The active component in milk thistle has been proven to down-regulate cancer-causing genes* so malignancy cell don't multiply effectively.

What does *Milk Thistle* do for the Liver Organ?

Milk thistle is among the best natural herbs for liver organ detox, since it has such a robust influence on liver organ function. It helps to:

- Reduce inflammation.

- Stabilize membranes in the liver.

- Increase glutathione production.

- Increase Superoxide Dismutase.

- And decrease liver organ tumor cellular division.

It also will protect your liver organ from the harm created as it detoxifies toxins. *Milk thistle* even escalates the success time of individuals with alcohol-related liver organ cirrhosis!

Milk thistle has virtually identical results on our two detoxification organs. It's our top choice for natural kidney and liver organ detox.

Marshmallow Root

Marshmallow originates from a Greek term meaning *"to heal."* It generates mucilage when you ingest it and has typically been used to take care of sore throats. *It is anti-inflammatory, antibacterial and antifungal.* Luckily, this herb will do great things for our kidneys and liver organ as well.

What does Marshmallow root do for the Kidneys?

One potential concern that individuals have is developing kidney stone.

How will you flush your kidneys to assist in preventing them?

By firmly taking herbs which have a diuretic impact. Diuretics can boost the amount of urine you produce and flush out particles from the kidneys with it. Marshmallow underlying can become a diuretic to help you execute a natural kidney cleanse.

What does Marshmallow root do for the liver organ?

Marshmallow root has ***polysaccharides*** that assist in wound therapeutic due to its high antioxidant capacity. Liver organ bile ducts may become damaged as time passes. Marshmallow root functions to soothe this harm. Actually, it stimulates the creation of our epithelial cell. They are the cell that lies within our organs and ducts. Having a solid, healthy bile duct can better help your liver organ detox.

One additional benefits of marshmallow is its capability to bind to toxins. Binding toxins and ushering them out of the body before they can create harm. In other words, we love this root for liver organ and kidney cleansing.

Parsley

This green herb is a lot greater than a garnish on your plate at a restaurant! *It really is filled with flavonoids, vitamins, nutrients, and antioxidants.* Parsley has some powerful kidney and liver organ detoxification properties we may take advantage of.

What does parsley do for the kidneys?

Parsley is another fantastic herb to help us prevent kidney stone since it is a diuretic. When analyzed against other chemicals, parsley reduced kidney stone the most. Not merely did the scale and quantity of stone significantly decrease, however the kidney cells was also healthier. Parsley is a robust natural kidney cleanse supplement.

What does parsley do for the liver organ?

Parsley is known as a "bitter" herb. Bitter herbal products can help excite your release of bile, assisting the liver cleansing. Parsley also really helps to produce glutathione which helps protect your liver organ from harm.

Parsley can also help lower your blood sugar levels, which can inflame the liver organ if they're too high. It can beneficially protect your liver organ by decreasing inflammatory liver organ enzymes.

Much like marshmallow, parsley can help bind onto and remove toxins from the body.

Parsley's diuretic and protective functions make it a particularly good kidney detoxification herb that also offers benefits for our liver organ!

Gynostemma

This herb has been used for a large number of years. It's been nicknamed "poor man's ginseng" since one of its chemical substance constituents is equivalent to Korean ginseng. It's best for the disease fighting capability and supports energy. It also helps our liver organ and kidney cleansing process.

What does Gynostemma do for the kidneys?

When our organs are injured from contact with toxins, an activity called fibrosis may appear. That is when our cell create scar tissue formation rather than healthy tissue. Scar tissue formation doesn't function like healthy tissues and inhibits our kidney's capability to detoxification optimally. High degrees of fibrosis can result in the increased loss of kidney function completely. *Gynostemma can impact the genes inside our kidneys to help produce healthy, well-functioning cells and reduce fibrosis.*

What does Gynostemma do for the liver organ?

Gynostemma gets the same fibrosis lowering results in the liver organ as it does on the kidney. Scar tissue formation eventually ends up being solid and unyielding, stopping your liver organ from working properly. One research showed that liver organ tissues can slim out, and severe liver organ fibrosis can be reduced by 33% in less than eight weeks! Healthy tissues can help your liver cleansing at its best capacity.

It also affects your genes involved with liver cancer cell development and has been proven to inhibit them from multiplying, which would help protect you from liver organ cancer.

Gynostemma is a robust anti-inflammatory for our intestines as well. The intestines will be the next thing in your liver organ detox. The liver organ dumps its harmful toxins into this part of your drainage system to be studied from the body. *Gynostemma will triple responsibility by assisting our kidneys, liver organ, and intestines.* This makes it one of our favorites to improve your natural detoxification.

Beetroot

Beetroot is a lot more than the veggie you didn't like as a youngster. They've been consumed for a large number of years for their health advantages. Beets were within Egyptian pyramids back to the 3rd Dynasty. Even without knowing it, these were assisting their liver organ and kidneys cleansing by eating beets.

What does beetroot do for the kidneys?

Beetroot can boost your creation of nitric oxide. Nitric oxide dilates arteries which increases blood circulation. This additional blood circulation can help your kidneys better than whenever your blood flow is fixed.

The scarlet pigment of beetroot is named **betanin**. It can help reduce irritation and oxidative stress. Additionally, it may help protect your kidneys from harm.

Beetroot can also help protect your kidneys from being injured from antibiotics, which will often cause kidney failing. It can help to increase catalase, your own natural in-house antioxidant which is vital for effective kidney detoxification. Beetroot allows you to downregulate proinflammatory chemicals in the kidneys as well.

What does beetroot do for the liver organ?

Your liver organ is the body organ that protects you from foreign substances also known as *xenobiotics*. Xenobiotics include items you are most likely subjected to daily like pesticides, air pollution, and food chemicals.

They may be carcinogenic (cancer-causing) which means that your liver wants to cope with them immediately. However, they can still harm the liver organ as it neutralizes them. Beetroot really helps to boost your own natural antioxidants to safeguard the liver organ from harm. Problems for your DNA may also be reduced.

The process of getting gone these foreign substances is named phase II metabolism. The red pigment betanin helps quench the free radicals that are a byproduct of the cleansing pathway and make it better for all of us.

Beetroot is another plant that affects our genes. It can help downregulate the genes associated with liver malignancy.

Beetroot's protective pigment and gene influencing properties make it on top of our set of natural liver and kidney detox herbs.

Ginger

Ginger is the hottest spice in the world. We often use this pungent natural herb for nausea, but it's assisting your liver organ and kidneys detoxification as well.

What does ginger do for the kidneys?

Ginger can have a robust influence on your kidney cleansing capabilities!

It's been proven to:

- Raise the body's natural antioxidants in the kidneys.

- Lower inflammation.

- Help remove harmful toxins from the kidneys.

- Reduce fibrosis.

- Help create healthier kidney cells.

    This simple root herb is a powerhouse for kidney detox.

What does ginger do for the liver organ?

Ginger will not disappoint as it pertains to our liver organ detox either.

Experts aren't sure how ginger will do it, but it can impact our genes associated with producing body fat in the liver organ. It helps to avoid lipid storage space, which can help protect us from fatty liver organ disease. Having excess fat accumulate in the liver organ, prevents it from doing its 500 jobs properly. It leads to fibrosis and reduces the blood circulation to the liver organ, which greatly reduces detoxification.

Ginger reduces inflammation almost immediately ,it helps us produce our very own antioxidants.

Another benefit that applies to both our liver organ and kidneys, is protection from toxins. Cadmium can transform gene appearance and upregulate malignancy genes. Ginger reverses this and helps protect you from toxins.

Ginger is a simple, but powerful addition to your kidney and liver organ detox protocol.

Chapter 6

How to Detox Your Blood

How will you clean your blood?

Detox is a significant buzzword of the 21st century. From diet detoxes to cleansing, to blood detoxes, some various programs and techniques guarantee to help you cleanse and detoxify the body.

Ideally, once you perform one of the detoxes, you'll feel more vigorous. However, lots of such statements don't possess a great deal of research in it, especially when they forget the role your liver organ already takes on cleaning your blood.

So how exactly does your liver organ clean your blood?

The liver organ is one of your largest organs. It's essential in detoxifying the body.

Your liver organ:

- filters your blood.

- processes nutrients.

- removes toxins, like the byproducts from the break down of medications and alcohol.

Contained in your liver are a large number of lobules. These small areas filter system blood production, and to push out a toxin called bile to breakdown substances within you.

A number of the specific ways your liver organ breaks down harmful toxins include:

- changing ammonia to urea.

- processing and removing excess bilirubin, which is a waste material product of the break down of red blood vessels cells.

- producing disease fighting capability cells to remove bacteria and potential toxins and bacteria from your blood.

While your liver may be your primary blood filter, you have other filtering organs.

- Your lungs filter harmful substances in the air, such as toxins from tobacco smoke.

Your intestines destroy parasites and other unwanted organisms.

- Your kidneys filtration system filters excess harmful toxins and waste from your blood and releases them in your urine.

What to Know before taking any Herb

Many products on the marketplace advertise themselves as detox agents.

Detox Tea

Many health food stores and pharmacies sell detoxification teas created from a number of herbs. For example *dandelion and nettle leaf* that have diuretic properties. Other products, such as *senna leaf*, have a laxative impact.

As good as these teas may be, they probably haven't any better cleansing properties when compared to a **glass of green or black tea.**

Charcoal Beverages and Juices

Doctors have used activated charcoal for a long time to lessen intestinal absorption and effects of certain poisons.

Now, juice and drink manufacturers are adding levels of charcoal to beverages, encouraging to detoxify the body. They state the charcoal can bind to the harmful toxins in your intestinal system to lessen the degrees of dangerous substances that enter your blood.

However, there isn't any lot of research to aid the advantages of charcoal put into drinks. No technology confirms that charcoal's especially help in detoxifying your blood or keeping you healthy. Some individuals who consume these beverages say they feel better when they are doing, while others might not experience results.

The Mayo Clinic has more information on medications that interact or lose effectiveness when activated charcoal is taken orally. You must never take activated charcoal if you have a brief history of blood loss in the belly or colon, experienced recent surgery, or end up having indigestion. It is possible to overdose on activated charcoal. I recommend not taking activated charcoal orally without first speaking with your doctor.

The FDA will not approve or monitor activated charcoal or any other natural treatments.

Detox Diets

The idea of detox diets been around for many years. They usually contain a restrictive diet to cleanse your blood and typically promote weight loss. Detoxification diets usually eliminate chemicals such as:

- Alcohol.

- Caffeine.

- Gluten.

- red meat.

- refined sugars, among others.

Some cleansing diets can promote healthier eating. Others can be quite restrictive, such as juice detox or other diets that revolve around restrictions from any foods and beverages to help you get energy.

As your body can mainly flush out toxins alone, a restrictive diet program isn't necessary. A healthy diet, such as one which contains a lot of fruits, vegetables, liver organ, and whole grains, will help.

Safeguarding Your Liver

As a result of your liver being an important organ in cleaning your blood, you should do something to safeguard it. Luckily, many regular healthy practices can help keep your liver organ in form. Some tips are:

- ***Get vaccinated against Hepatitis A and B***: These conditions are viral infections that may damage your liver.

- ***Maintain a wholesome weight***: Carrying excess fat can donate to a disorder called non-alcoholic fatty liver organ disease. Eating a healthy diet and working out can help you keep up a wholesome weight.

- ***Don't share fine needles or use contaminated needles***: If you get tattoos or body piercings, enquire about the shop's cleaning practices to guarantee the needles aren't contaminated.

- ***Practice safe sex***: This minimises your dangers of sexually infections such as viral infections of hepatitis B or C.

- ***Follow the suggestions outlined on your medications***: This is also true whenever your medication's label says never to consume alcohol while taking it.

- ***Avoid excess alcohol***: Your liver filter your body systems and detoxifies alcoholic beverages with many other products. When there are too many alcoholic beverages in your blood, the surplus can scar tissue and destroy liver organ cells.

- ***Avoid using illicit drugs***: Your liver organ filters harmful byproducts from medication use. Chronic use can result in severe harm to your liver organ, especially when coupled with alcohol.

5 Fail-proof Herbs for Detoxifying Blood Naturally & their Preparations

The liver organ, your body's detoxifying organ, is continually filtering blood to remove any chemicals or toxins that may have finished up in your blood stream. How about producing a little help? Blood cleaning herbs eliminate harmful toxins from the lymph system, kidneys, and liver organ, ensuring real untainted blood circulates through the body to the many organs.

These five herbs are often available and work very well to purify your blood and support overall detoxification, thus promoting good health.

1. Burdock Root

Known because of its blood-cleansing properties, burdock is known as a premier pore and skin herb. It cleanses harmful toxins from your body by dealing with the liver organ and lymph system. Burdock is also known because of its diuretic properties and aids the kidneys in filtering harmful particles from the blood. Abundant with iron, this nourishing root is ideal for enriching the blood and strengthening the whole system.

How to use it:

Burdock can be taken in a variety of forms such as pills, liquid extracts, tinctures, or tea. As an edible root you will get it in the new produce portion of your neighborhood health store. Vaporize it with fresh vegetables or use in soups.

2. Dandelion

Packed with phytonutrients and a number of antioxidants, this herbal weed can eliminate toxins from your digestive system, and blood, and also scavenge free radicals.

Dandelion stimulates the liver organ and pancreas to grab harmful toxins from the blood and detoxify your blood.

How to use it:

The simplest way to take pleasure from the detoxifying advantages of dandelion is to brew a tea with fresh or dried out dandelion leaves, plants or root.

3. Reishi Mushroom

A Chinese tonic, this herb enhances the liver's cleansing process. *Reishi mushroom* is abundant with ganoderic acidity, which functions as an *antihistamine* and reduces swelling. It also boosts the utilization of oxygen in the blood, thus enriching it. *Triterpenes and ganodosterone* within this mushroom have antihepatotoxic properties and therefore guard the liver organ against damage. It has additionally been proven to regenerate liver organ cell in patients with severe hepatitis.

How to use it:

Boil 2tsp of dried out mushroom in a single cup of water. Simmer for just two to 3 minutes and drink once cool. You can even sprinkle powdered mushroom over your soups.

4. Basil

This culinary herb is most beneficial known because of its antibacterial and anti-inflammatory properties. Basil also offers an exceptional capability to purify your blood and removal of any harmful accumulation from the liver organ and kidneys. A fantastic diuretic, basil supports eliminating harmful toxins from your body via urine.

How exactly to use:

Squeeze 5 to 6 basil leaves and add it to your soups, salads, or pasta for a few extra flavor and detoxifying benefits. You can even make a natural tea by making 6 to 8 basil leaves in a glass of warm water.

5. Red Clover

These lilac blossoms are excellent blood purifiers that steadily work to improve any defect in the circulatory system. Besides, it enhances the blood flow by preventing the forming of clots. Red clover is also known because of its anti-tumor properties, and it is widely used by herbalists worldwide (Dr Sebi among others) as an anti-cancer treatment.

How exactly to use:

Steep a relaxing and detoxifying red clover tea by using 3 to 4 fresh blossoms or 1tsp of smashed dried flowers in a single cup of warm water for ten minutes. Drink once cool. You can even buy ready-to-go teabags and pills online.

www.ingramcontent.com/pod-product-compliance
Lightning Source LLC
Chambersburg PA
CBHW071126030426
42336CB00013BA/2216